How To Make Liposomal Vitamin C

Cheryl Hines

DEDICATION

I would not have thought to try making my own Liposomal Vitamin C had my father-in-law, Ross Hines, not told me of it in the first place.

Thanks, Dad

CONTENTS

ACKNOWLEDGMENTS 7

DISCLAIMER 9

Important – Please read 10

General advice... 11

Introduction 12

Why make your own Liposomal Vitamin C? 13

Commercial vs Homemade LET Vitamin C................. 13

FAQs 15

What You Will Need 19

Procedure for large batch................................20

Procedure for small batch 22

Procedure for using ascorbic acid and sodium
bicarbonate (baking soda) 24

Step-by-step directions 26

Final thoughts 31

Troubleshooting & Tips 32

Test for percent encapsulation 34

Directions for use 35

Cost break down (as of 4/2014) 36

ABOUT THE AUTHOR 37

ACKNOWLEDGMENTS

To my family: Mark, my patient husband, and nine beautiful kids. Thanks for letting me experiment on you and being willing to taste and try. And for pretending it all tasted "good". I love you all.

To Mr. Brooks Bradley: the father of homemade LET and champion of the weekend scientist. This book couldn't be without your untiring scientific curiosity which made this modern advancement in technology obtainable to the casual scientist like me. My sincere gratitude goes to you.

DISCLAIMER

This guide is intended to provide helpful and informative material on the subjects addressed in the publication. It is sold with the understanding that the author and publishers are not engaged in rendering medical, health or any other kind of personal professional services in this book. The reader should consult his or her medical, health, or other competent professional before adopting any of the suggestions in this book or drawing inferences from it.

The author specifically disclaims all responsibility for any liability, loss, or risk, personal or otherwise, which is incurred as a consequence, directly or indirectly, of the use and application of any of the contents in this book.

To repeat: If you are ill, please do not hesitate to consult a qualified health care provider.

Important – Please read

Dear Reader:

If you or your loved one is seriously ill, I urge you to see your trusted medical professional for advice. I am not a doctor or health care professional and as such will not prescribe. I only offer this small book to educate and entertain.

I expect that anyone reading this book will take responsibility for their own health.

Allergy warning: Those who have corn allergies might have an allergic reaction to ascorbic acid or sodium ascorbate as some brands are derived from corn. If you are allergic to corn, please check your labels.

General advice

LET Vitamin C is a fabulous discovery but it must not be used like a Band-Aid. It can and does work wonders but for it to work long term, please consider making other supportive lifestyle changes such as reducing stress (#1), adding more and more fresh vegetables to your diet, getting more sleep, fresh air and daily movement, etc.

Holistic attitude is all about assisting the body to heal itself, not ignore its innate ability to get well. We don't want to start to use alternative treatments the same way traditional medicine uses drugs and surgery. So, I would never use or recommend anyone take *large* doses of liposomal vitamin C on a long term basis.

A licensed naturopath friend of mine cautioned me to not take megadose LET vitamin C long term (or any medical treatment, for that matter) but use it like any short term treatment - to get the job done. As good as it is for you, acid is acid. The body has to balance the pH by taking calcium out of the bloodstream. If it isn't there it will take from bones and tissue. Our body can handle short term imbalance in order to get well. But erosion of our bones and tissues might be the result if carried on long term.

A suggested protocol: During acute treatments where you are aggressively treating an illness, take a day off every 5 or 7 days. This way your body has a chance to work on its own – build its own defense system.

Introduction

Nothing new under the sun...

Let me first acknowledge freely that the basic information contained in this short guide is gleaned from several dozens of articles and a handful of books. It is my hope that this will save you time having it all distilled into one place

The man who deserves credit for pioneering homemade LET (liposomal encapsulation technology) is Brooks Bradley. While there have been others who have contributed, you will almost always find that they reference Bradley's work. The basic process is based on his suggestions. As the process evolved, he continued to make comments making it possible for people like you and me to take charge of our own health using LET Vitamin C.

Therefore you have in your hands a book which is the result of dozens of hours of personal trials and tweaking on how to make Liposomal Encapsulated Technology (LET) Vitamin C (ascorbic acid*) at home.

> Note: Making your own liposomal Vitamin C is fairly simple and since the ingredients as well as the final formula are non-toxic, there is room for slight variations in amounts and ingredients.

How-to book not a *why*-to book

I will not be discussing the benefits of taking mega doses of ascorbic acid. I assume that you know that Vitamin C is nature's best kept secret for long life and perfect health but you want to know one of the most absorbable ways to take it.

For those interested in learning more, I list several on my website: http://simplefrugal.com/vitamin-c-resources/

12

* For the purposes of this short guide, I will use the term vitamin C and ascorbic acid interchangeably. Yes, I am aware that there is a difference and is noted in the FAQs.

Why make your own Liposomal Vitamin C?

While regular Vitamin C is relatively inexpensive and easy to find/purchase, commercially made lipospheric or liposomal Vitamin C products are costly in the amounts suggested for healing therapies or even for health maintenance. In my research, I found that the least expensive form was a dollar per 1000 mg dose. In therapeutic amounts that would quickly become cost prohibitive.

At the end of this short book I give a breakdown of how much it costs to make home-made Liposomal Vitamin C. Suffice it to say, I love to do things myself if it is cost effective and relatively simple. At 10¢ per ounce (roughly 900 mg of available ascorbic acid), I can say it is very cost effective.

As you will read in a bit, it is relatively simple to make, too. Even my 10 year old makes it. But it is important to follow the instructions closely. **Stirring is particularly important** as it assures that the lecithin encapsulates the sodium ascorbate as much as possible. The more thoroughly it is encapsulated, the more absorbable it is.

Commercial vs Homemade LET Vitamin C

I can't claim this process makes 100% encapsulated LET Vitamin C. I don't have access to laboratories or equipment to test encapsulation. I am trusting a process offered by a man who knew what he was doing – Brooks Bradley.

Others who have made homemade LET vitamin C have used crude test, like the one I include later in this book which indicate anywhere from 50% to 85% encapsulation. By my calculations, that still provides an excellent uptake of vitamin C and keeps the cost very low.

I don't compare my homemade version to the commercial version anymore than I would compare my homemade herbal medicines to the commercially sold standardized versions. I just know they work the way they are supposed to for me.

Since ascorbic acid is a relatively harmless compound, you can't over do it. You might get loose stools but that just means to back down. Take a day off. Then use less next time.

FAQs

How do you know if your liposomal Vitamin C is encapsulated?

I have included a test to help you determine just how encapsulated your finished product is (credit goes to Brooks Bradley).

In any case, LET (liposomal encapsulation technology) is still a very new science. Even experts say there is no way to exactly determine whether liposomes are present and if they are, are they stable (won't "unencapsulate").

Even at 50% encapsulation, it is estimated that one is getting at least as much sodium ascorbate as if a patient were to receive it in an IV. This is because the lecithin bubble is by far more friendly to the cells than non-LET ascorbic acid.

So, even if my procedure resulted in only 50% efficient encapsulation, it is still very effective.

If LET Vitamin C is unstable, how much should I make?

Because homemade liposomal ascorbic acid is relatively unstable, it will break down making more and more ascorbic acid unencapsulated. I recommend you make only as much LET Vitamin C as you might use in a week but plan to refrigerate it.

For example, for my large family I would make 3 large (48oz) batches at a time as we would take anywhere from 1 to 3 ounces at a time – each! We would go through a quart a day during cold season.

I have included procedures for a small approximately 16oz batch for one person for a few days.

Why Sodium Ascorbate? Why can't I just use ascorbic acid?

I use sodium ascorbate as it is the same buffered form of

ascorbic acid which physicians use when they give ascorbic acid/Vitamin C intravenously. It is also what you will find in commercially available liposomal Vitamin C.

The reason: Straight pharmaceutical grade ascorbic acid is too acidic (4.2pH) to use for our purposes. If you take straight ascorbic acid into the blood stream, it would cause the body to need to neutralize the pH by taking calcium among other things from your body to balance it, namely from your bones and teeth.

Since the body's pH level is tightly regulated at a slightly alkaline 7.35 to 7.45, you want to try to make sure anything you introduce directly into the blood stream of *similar* pH. Sodium ascorbate is a buffered version which eliminates this problem. It is close to 6.9 pH which is slightly acidic but manageable.

I am aware that my readers may have some ascorbic acid on hand and rather than waste it, I am including a procedure that allows you to use your ascorbic acid by making your own sodium ascorbate acid using sodium bicarbonate (baking soda). See that section.

Can I use any other mineral ascorbates like calcium ascorbate, magnesium ascorbate, zinc ascorbate, etc?

According to Dr Thomas Levy M.D. he cautions against using any form of ascorbate *except* sodium ascorbate. The reason being that in the quantity of liposomal form of ascorbate we use, the mineral would reach a toxic level in your blood stream. He only recommends sodium ascorbate.

I want to use sunflower lecithin instead of soy lecithin, is that OK?

Yes, you can use sunflower lecithin. For those using sunflower lecithin, keep in mind the finished product will look different from the soy lecithin version. I have been told it looks like a highly creamed coffee (beige) colored.

How much liposomal Vitamin C should I take?

This is a book on *how to make* liposomal Vitamin C not

how to take it, thus I cannot make any prescriptions or recommendations. Please read more about the therapeutic benefits of liposomal Vitamin C on the internet or Primal Panacea by Dr. Thomas.

My pet is ill. Can I give it to it?

I have no experience with this but several readers have said they have used it successfully.

Oops! I might have not added enough water or sodium ascorbate or lecithin. What can I do to fix it?

First of all, lecithin is a very nutritious food in and of itself, so no problem there. Sodium ascorbate is non toxic and will only cause a loose stool if you take too much.

I have learned that there is no need to be exact as long as you follow the 3 to 1 volume ratio of lecithin to ascorbic acid, whether it's 3 tablespoons lecithin to 1 tablespoon Vitamin C or ¾ cup to ¼ cup.

Even the water isn't terribly critical as long as you have enough to dissolve the ascorbic acid and melt the lecithin granules. It simply results in a thicker or thinner end product.

I have seen "recipes" for making liposomal Vitamin C that use a third to half the water that I use. Their results are thicker and more like egg yolk in consistency.

Why do you use the term Vitamin C and ascorbic acid synonymously? They are not the same.

You are correct. They are not the same. Vitamin C refers to the compound of nutrients, which **includes** ascorbic acid, that are present in many fruits and vegetables, namely citrus fruits of all kinds.

Ascorbic acid is the isolated part of Vitamin C. It is the active part which has been used effectively in treatment of colds among other things.

Some will argue that you cannot call what I make (and I will note that even the commercial variety) liposomal Vitamin C when in fact we use ascorbic acid or sodium ascorbate, as the case may be.

While I might literally go through my book and change it all, I hope that you can overlook the term.

Should I be concerned about making the solution in the stainless steel ultrasound tub? Won't it give off molecules of nickel into my solution?

An excellent point. It is a fact that over time, the inner stainless steel tub will "cavitate" or give off miniscule amounts of metal. This is why many will make homemade LET Vitamin C in beakers or thin walled glass containers within the ultrasonic unit.

Put the glass container into the unit and fill the unit with enough water to go to fill line. You still have to stir as recommended.

I am concerned about taking that much sodium. Is there another way to take this without using sodium ascorbate?

While Dr Levy doesn't recommend it, you are free to use regular ascorbic acid. Just use it on a short term basis. Keep in mind that ascorbic acid will acidify your blood and cause other long-term problems. FYI: A one ounce "dose" of homemade LET vitamin C contains approximately 100mg sodium.

What You Will Need

Ingredients:
- Lecithin granules, non GMO Soy or sunflower*
- Sodium ascorbate powder
- Distilled water
- non-aluminum baking soda (optional)

Equipment and supplies:
- 2 one quart canning jars + lids for storage
- 1 pint jar + lid for mixing ascorbic acid powder
- Dry and liquid measuring cups
- Blender (we use a Vitamix)
- Ultrasonic jewelry cleaner, large for 48oz.
- Plastic ladle, straws or plastic spoon for stirring (I get extras at fast food restaurants). **Nothing metal.**

*You can use liquid lecithin but use half the amount.

For suggestions and a list of where I get my equipment and supplies, see my resources page:
http://simplefrugal.com/vitamin-c-resources/

Procedure for large batch

Approx. 48 oz. (48 grams sodium ascorbate)

Use the following proportions:

¾ cup (100g) lecithin granules
30 oz (890ml) distilled water
¼ cup (48g) Sodium Ascorbate powder
12 oz (350ml) distilled water

Pour 30 oz. (890ml) distilled water that is at least room temperature (can be warmer) into the VitaMix or large blender (I prefer my Vitamix simply because it has an ultra low stirring speed). I have made a permanent line on my blender at the water line.

Turn Vitamix on lowest setting.

Measure and add lecithin granules to the water stirring in the Vitamix.

Stir on low till the lecithin is melted – this can take 5 - 10 minutes depending on the temperature of the water. Will look like a creamy bright, lemon yellow color.

Meanwhile, in the pint jar, pour 12 oz (350 ml) distilled water and **sodium ascorbate** powder. Put on lid and shake till all is dissolved.

Next, pour the ascorbate solution into lecithin mixture while still blending. Let it blend a minute or so. Some suggest you blend for 5 or more minutes in to help with the homogenization.

Pour lecithin/Vitamin C solution into the ultrasonic cleaner. If you are using a smaller unit, pour to the max fill line.

Set for longest cycle on your machine. Mine has 480 second cycle which translates to 8 minutes. Some units have different times, so you might have to figure out different cycles if your machine does shorter cycles. The idea is to homogenize for approximately 30 minutes.

Stir fairly often using a plastic soup ladle, straws or spoon. Stirring keeps the lecithin moving till it has "encapsulated" the sodium ascorbate. The more you stir, the more homogenized is the final solution.

Finally, ladle/pour into labeled storage jar. Store in refrigerator. Can be used right away. It can store in fridge for up to a week.

**Note to users of sunflower lecithin: My readers who have used sunflower lecithin say that the final product is more the color of creamed coffee.

Procedure for small batch

Approximately 16 oz. (16 g sodium ascorbate)

Use the following proportions:

> **10 oz (300ml) distilled water**
> **¼ cup (33g) lecithin granules**
> **4 oz (120ml) distilled water**
> **1 tablespoon +1 teaspoon (16g) sodium ascorbate**

Pour 10 oz (300ml) distilled water that is at least room temperature(can be warmer) into the VitaMix or large blender (I prefer my Vitamix simply because it has an ultra low stirring speed). I have made a permanent line on my blender at the water line.

Turn Vitamix on lowest setting.

Measure and add **lecithin granules** to the water stirring in the Vitamix.

Stir on low till the lecithin is homogenized – this can take 5 - 10 minutes depending on the temperature of the water. Will look like a creamy bright, lemon yellow color.

Meanwhile, in the pint jar, pour 4 oz (120 ml) distilled water and **sodium ascorbate** powder. Put on lid and shake till all is dissolved.

Next, pour the ascorbate solution into lecithin mixture while still blending. Let it blend a minute or so. Some suggest you blend for 5 or more minutes in to help with the homogenization.

Pour lecithin/Vitamin C solution into the ultrasonic cleaner. If you are using a smaller unit, pour to the max fill line.

Set for longest cycle on your machine. Mine has 480 second cycle which translates to 8 minutes. Some units have different times, so you might have to figure out different cycles if your machine does shorter cycles. The idea is to homogenize for approximately 30 minutes.

Stir fairly often using a plastic ladle, straw or spoon. Stirring keeps the lecithin moving till it has "encapsulated" the sodium ascorbate. The more you stir, the more homogenized is the final solution.

Finally - ladle/pour into labeled storage jar. Store in refrigerator. Can be used right away. It can store in fridge for up to a week.

**Note to users of sunflower lecithin: My readers who have used sunflower lecithin say that the final product is more the color of creamed coffee.

Procedure for using ascorbic acid and sodium bicarbonate (baking soda)

Approximately 16 oz batch

These are the original Brooks Bradley ingredients list. I have added them here for those who want to use ascorbic acid instead of sodium ascorbate. The main difference between this formula and the sodium ascorbate version I demonstrate in the book is that with this version, you are doing the buffering yourself. FYI—Sodium ascorbate is made by reacting ascorbic acid with bicarbonate of soda. Using sodium ascorbate in my other procedures just saves this step.

3 level tablespoons Lecithin granules
1 level tablespoon Ascorbic acid powder
1 level tablespoon plus 2 level teaspoons sodium bicarbonate, aluminum free (Bob's Red Mill brand, for example)*
Distilled water, gallon, to be measured

- Pour **8 oz distilled water** that is room temperature into the VitaMix or large blender (I prefer my Vitamix simply because it has an ultra low stirring speed). I have made a permanent line on my blender at the water line.
- Turn Vitamix on lowest setting.
- Measure and add lecithin granules to the water stirring in the Vitamix.
- Stir on low till the lecithin is homogenized. This can take 5 - 10 minutes depending on the temperature of the water. Will look like a creamy bright, lemon yellow color.
- Meanwhile, in a quart jar, pour **2 oz. distilled water** and ascorbic acid powder. Stir till all is dissolved.
- In a pint jar, add the soda to **2 ounces water**. Put on lid and shake till dissolved.

- Now, SLOWLY dribble the soda water into ascorbic acid solution while stirring. It will bubble furiously. Keep stirring and dribbling till the bubbling stops. Once it has stopped the soda will have reacted to the ascorbic acid and the result is buffered sodium ascorbate!

- Next, pour the ascorbate solution into lecithin mixture while still blending. Let it blend a minute or so. Some suggest you blend for 5 or more minutes in to help with the homogenization.

- Pour lecithin/Vitamin C solution into the ultrasonic cleaner. If you are using a smaller unit, pour to the max fill line.

- Set for 480 second cycle and turn on (480 seconds translates to 8 minutes). My large ultrasonic cleaner has cycles from 90, 180, 240, 360, and 480 seconds. Some units have different times, so you might have to figure out different cycles if your machine does shorter cycles. The idea is to homogenize for approximately 30 minutes.

- Stir fairly often using a plastic ladle or spoon. Stirring keeps the lecithin moving till it has "encapsulated" the sodium ascorbate. The more you stir, the more homogenized is the final solution. (Red blur is a straw which we used while doing the demonstration.)

- Finally - ladle/pour into labeled storage jar. Store in refrigerator. Can be used right away. It can store in fridge for up to a week.

*Many are concerned about the sodium when we add it to buffer. The amount I suggest here is based on the "recipe" widely available on the internet. It is the amount needed to completely buffer the acid.

Step-by-step directions

Demonstrating the large batch

1. Pour 30 oz (890ml) **distilled water** that is at least room temperature into the VitaMix or large blender (I prefer my Vitamix simply because it has an ultra low stirring speed). I have made a permanent line on my blender at the water line.

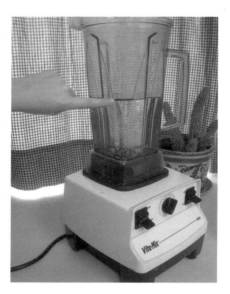

2. Set Vitamix (or blender) on lowest setting and turn it on.

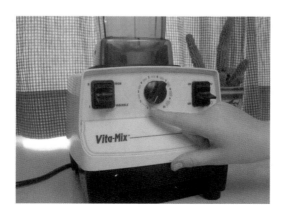

3. As the water is stirring, measure and add ¾ cup (100g) **lecithin granules** (using soy lecithin for this demonstration).

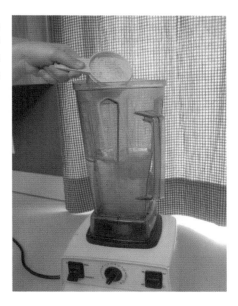

4. Continue stirring on low till the lecithin is homogenized – this can take about 5 - 10 minutes depending on the temperature of the water. I store my water in the house so it is room temp. Will look like a creamy bright, lemon yellow color (or beige if you are using sunflower lecithin).

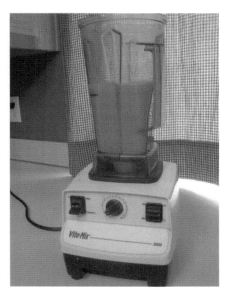

5. Meanwhile, in the pint jar, pour 12 oz (355 ml) distilled water and ¼ cup (58g) **sodium ascorbate** powder. Put on lid and shake till all is dissolved.

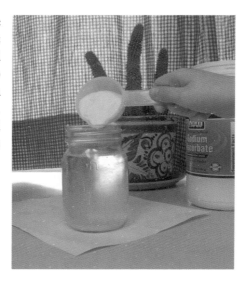

6. Next, pour the ascorbate solution into lecithin mixture while still blending. Let it blend a minute or so. Some suggest you blend for 5 or more minutes in to help with the homogenization.

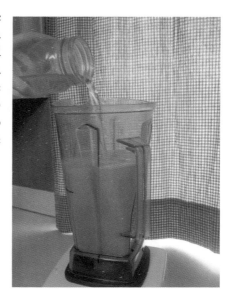

7. Pour lecithin/Vitamin C solution into the ultrasonic cleaner. If you are using a smaller unit, pour to the max fill line. The solution will have foam on top.

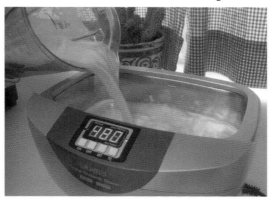

8. Set for longest cycle on your machine. Mine has 480 second cycle which translates to 8 minutes. Some units have different times, so you might have to figure out different cycles if your machine does shorter cycles. The idea is to homogenize for approximately 30 minutes.

9. **Stir fairly often** using a plastic ladle (our new preferred method) or straws (as pictured). **The more consistently you stir, the more homogenized is the final solution**.

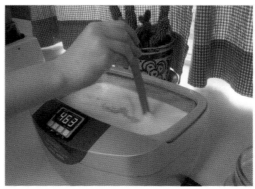

10. When the machines turns off, reset for 480 seconds and turn on again, stirring as before. Do this for 4 cycles or 32 minutes. Foam will be pretty much all gone. Finished product has somewhat watery consistency.

11. Finally - ladle/pour into labeled storage jar. Store in refrigerator.

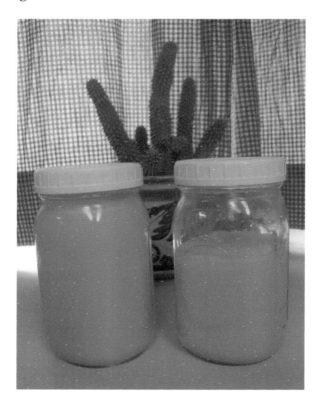

Can be used right away. Stores at room temperature for up to 4 days or in fridge for up to a week.

Actual color of finished product varies. It is more creamy lemon yellow when using soy lecithin or beige, creamed-coffee colored if using sunflower lecithin.

Final thoughts

I hope you found this helpful. Did I cover the subject of how to make your own liposomal Vitamin C well? I welcome your feedback. Did I leave something out?

Keep in mind I am not a scientist so this was not treated from that point of view. It is the result of my wide research and reading, then application of what I learned.

In any case, contact me at: http://simplefrugal.com to give me your thoughts. I will consider adding any useful information to the next revision of this book.

Troubleshooting & Tips

There is a darker layer on the bottom of the jar – what is it?

This layer is actually lecithin which didn't encapsulate during the stirring process. It just means you need to spend more time consistently stirring while it is being "zapped".

Is there a way to shorten the stirring process?

Not really. The stirring is critical to the encapsulation process. At first we used straws or plastic spoons. Later we found that a plastic soup ladle did the trick better than the straws.

The jars "leak" even if I tighten them – what's with that?

Lecithin has an odd way of making water thin out and leak around the jar lids. This is normal.

The taste is salty. How can I make it more palatable?

To make it more palatable, take in orange juice or Tang – whatever helps to get it down. Many of my kids just swig it down. Has a sort of soapy taste that some get used to.

I heard that the final product should be thick like egg yolk not watery.

One reader heard that it was not "good" unless it was thickened or viscous when properly processed. After investigating this I found that the thickness depends on how much water is added during the process. The amount of water added doesn't seem as critical in terms of how the final product works in your body. I tested several amounts of water, resulting in thicker final products and found that they worked as well as my original more watery instructions.

Use a timer and keep stirring

Making liposomal Vitamin C is not difficult at all but is it very time consuming. Monitoring the ultrasonic time can be tedious. We use a timer that sounds off when the machine stops "buzzing".

My final product is very watery. I thought it is supposed to be thick, like the commercial product.

I have read all over the internet and tried many versions of this formula. I will be the first to admit mine is not the only way to make liposomal vitamin C. Some use one third the water that I use and their result is rather thick like egg yolk.

What I found that is critical is as follows:

- Get the ratio of lecithin to ascorbate – 3 to 1.
- Make sure to completely dissolve the ascorbate in water before adding it to the lecithin.
- Agitate in jewelry cleaner for anywhere from 10 to 30 minutes. The variation seems to have to do with the depth of the solution in the machine. Some suggest keeping the amount shallow – no more than two inches and agitate for 10 minutes. I prefer to agitate my solution for 24 to 30 minutes at max fill.

Test for percent encapsulation

The following is a direct quotation by Brooks Bradley, the grandfather of homemade liposomal encapsulation technology (LET):

Brooks Bradley's simple test to gauge LET efficiency of a liposomal Vitamin C solution:

1) Pour 4 ounces of the finished LET Vitamin C into a 12oz container.

2) Add 1/4 teaspoon of sodium bicarbonate into 1 oz of distilled water, stirring well.

3) Pour the sodium bicarbonate solution into the LET Vitamin C mixture, stirring.

Results: If the resulting foam reaction line from this mixture is .5" or less you will have approximately a 50% encapsulation rate of the raw ascorbic acid nanoparticles. If the foam is 3/8" or less you will have approximately 60% encapsulation. If the foam is 1/8" thick or less, you will have around 75% encapsulation.

Foam occurs when the unencapsulated Vit C reacts with the sodium bicarbonate which is added to produce sodium ascorbate. The liposome encapsulated Vit C will not react. Thus, the less foam, the more Vit C is encapsulated and the more efficient went your process. By the way, this test solution should not be discarded as it is still valuable as a medicinal! The formed sodium ascorbate is a very useable form of Vitamin C.

Source:
http://www.vitamincfoundation.org/forum/viewtopic.php?f=20&t=7499&start=60

Directions for use

I used to make recommendations based on what my family and I had done after hundreds of batches with no ill effects. But I have been advised to not suggest any doses.

I encourage you to learn more about this on your own. I offer equipment suggestions as well as several resources on my site at: http://simplefrugal.com/vitamin-c-resources/

There is nothing so powerful as self education. Take charge of your own health.

Cost break down (as of 4/2014)

Feel free to find your own brands of lecithin and sodium ascorbate. Here are those I use which I find on Amazon.

NOW foods 10# Lecithin $85 at Amazon
I use approximately 3.5 oz lecithin per portion
1 0# equals 45 portions (160 /3.5 = 45.7)
$85 divided by 45 = $1.89 per recipe portion

NOW Foods 3 # Sodium Ascorbate $45 at Amazon
I use ¼ cup (2 oz) sodium ascorbate per portion
3# equals 60 portions (3 x 16 = 48; 48 / 2 = 24)
$45 divided by 24 = $1.88 per recipe portion

$1.89 + $1.88 = $3.77
$3.77 divided by 48 one ounce doses is **8¢ per dose** (approximately 1000 mg of sodium ascorbate)

That's a far cry from the $1 per packet commonly available.

ABOUT THE AUTHOR

Cheryl Hines is wife to Mark and mother of nine beautiful children and, at the time of this writing, grandma of three! You'll often find her "messing around" in the kitchen, baking bread from scratch, learning gluten free baking, and combining home remedies to help keep her family well. Her pet passion is to find ways to simplify and do it herself. She often teases that after two years in college, she is a career student at the University of Hard Knocks. As a result, she has discovered hundreds of tricks and hacks to simplify life.

Catch her at her "home" at **http://simplefrugal.com** where she shares her latest insights!

While visiting why not get updates and freebies when you sign up on the SimpleFrugal Family list, too.

Made in the USA
Lexington, KY
29 July 2014